OVERCOMING MENTAL HEALTH ISSUES

Realistic Ways to Psychological Well-being

Innocent Onunkwo

DEDICATION

This book is dedicated to all medical
personnels and care-givers

CONTENTS

INTRODUCTION

Humans are the greatest of all living things based on what their brains can think, take, process and execute. This gives them an edge over all living creatures, and the ability to manipulate every living and nonliving things.

Individuals can think, feel and behave differently, and an abnormality in any of these brings about the issues of mental health. World health organisation (WHO) described mental health as a state of mental well-being that enables people to cope with the stresses of life, realize their abilities, learn well and work well, and contribute to their community.

Since the brain controls what happens in the body, the psychological well-being of an individual will enable him or her to cope with stress, achieve his or her dreams, and as well, contribute his or her quota in solving human and existential problems.

There are simple and realistic ways to a good mental health state and to stay psychologically well even in the midst of unfavorable happenings and uncertainties, and they have been highlighted and well-explained in this book.

MUSIC

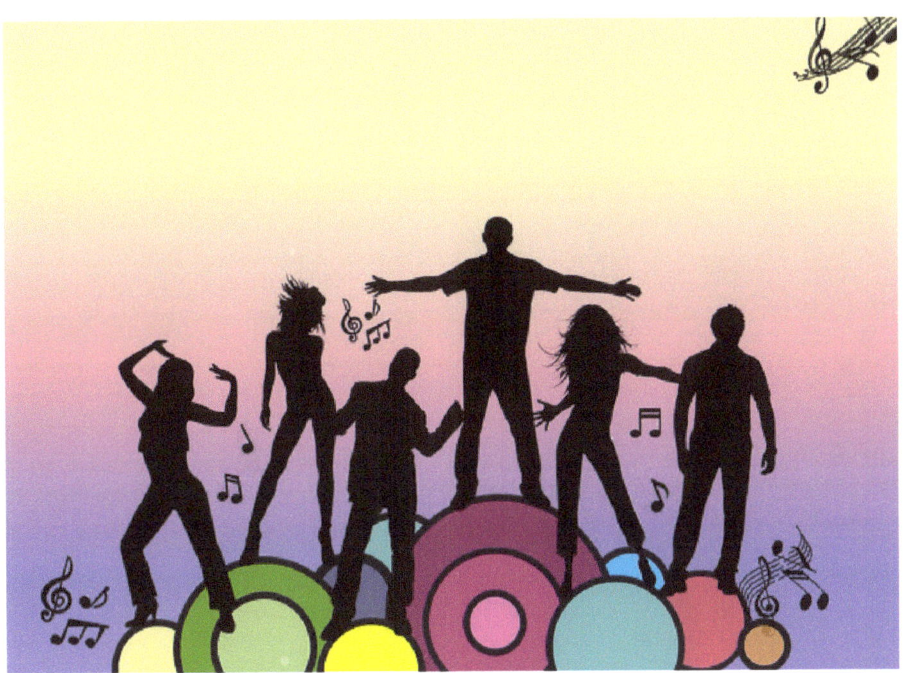

The relation of music (good songs and sounds) to mental well-being cannot be overemphasized. Music reduces stress by generating good and happy hormone. Good music make you think, feel and behave better. There are motivational, inspirational, happy, chilling, energetic songs and so on that can one can use to tackle mental health issues and improved psychological wellness, and they are just a click away.

Activity:

Create music playlists in your favourite streaming platform and add up songs that make you happy and feel motivated, develop the habit of listening to them more often. Sometimes, go to music shows and dance to the tunes.

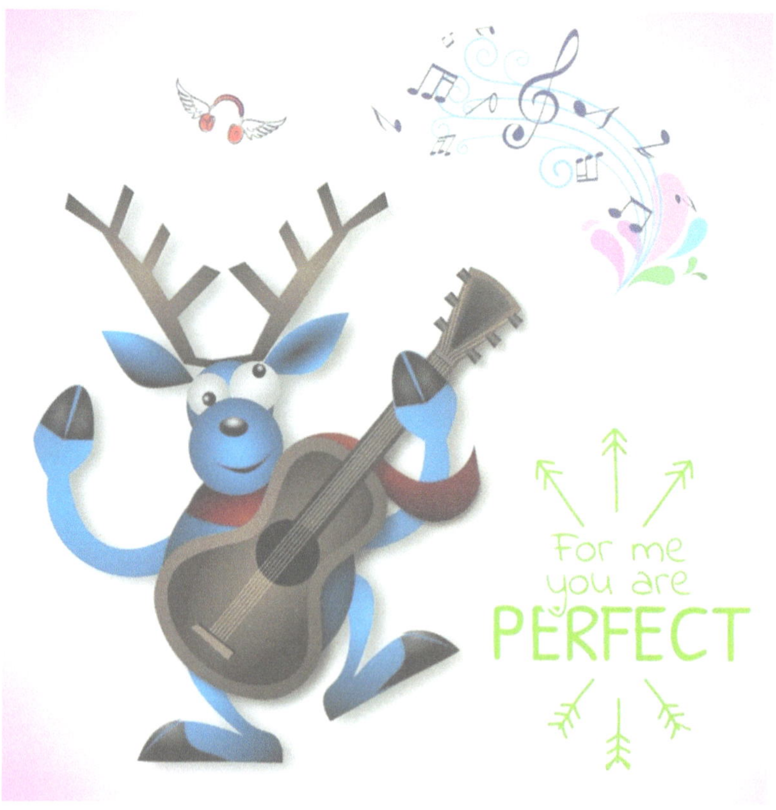

EXERCISE

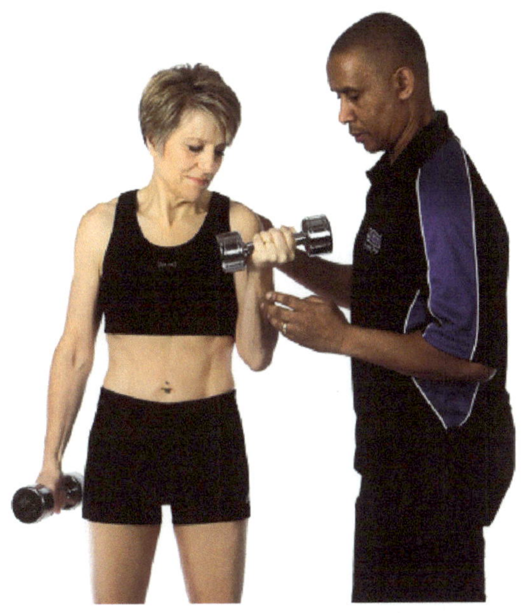

The relation of music (good songs and sounds) to mental well-being cannot be overemphasized. Music reduces stress by generating good and happy hormone. Good music make you think, feel and behave better. There are motivational, inspirational, happy, chilling, energetic songs and so on that can one can use to tackle mental health issues and improved psychological wellness, and they are just a click away.

Activity:

Engage yourself in simple daily exercise that has to do with stretching your body; and when you have a luxury of time, visit the gym.

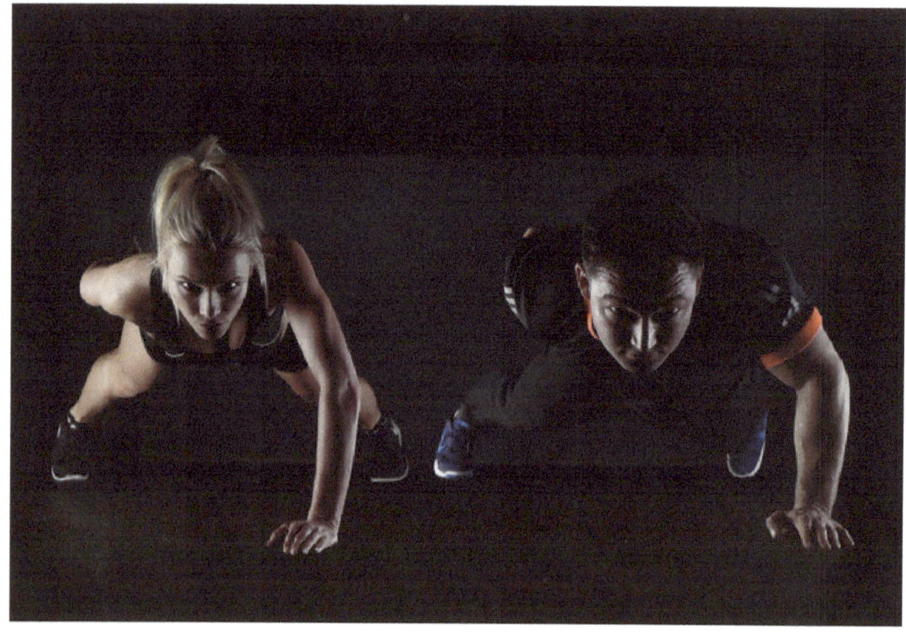

WORK PRINCIPLE

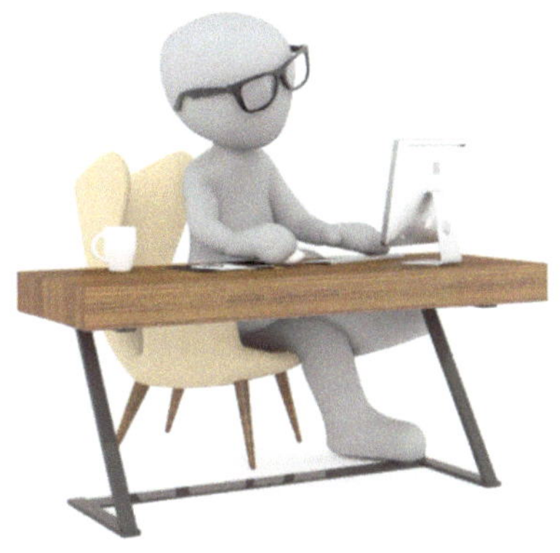

Work requires a lot of energy from one's system. One may exhaust all the energy in his/her body, if one doesn't apply principle, caution and restraint while working, and this can lead to a mental health challenge. Overworking one's brain can cause brain issues that may affect one's psychological well-being, as well as other parts of the body.

Activity:

Know the kind of job you can cope with and know when you're tired, as well as when to stop working.

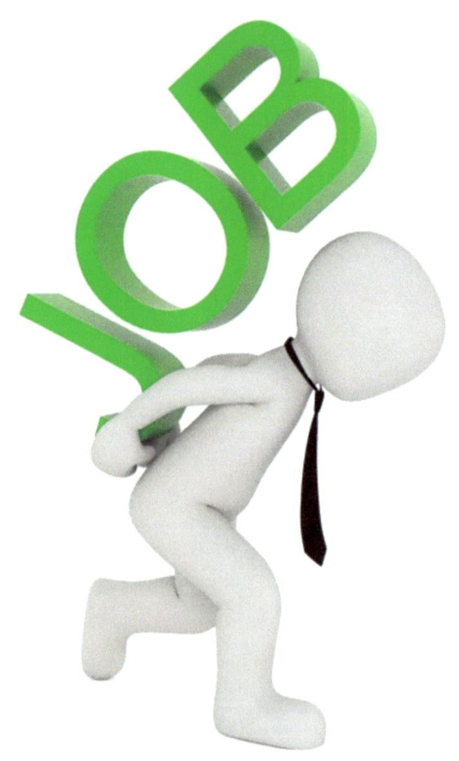

TIME MANAGEMENT

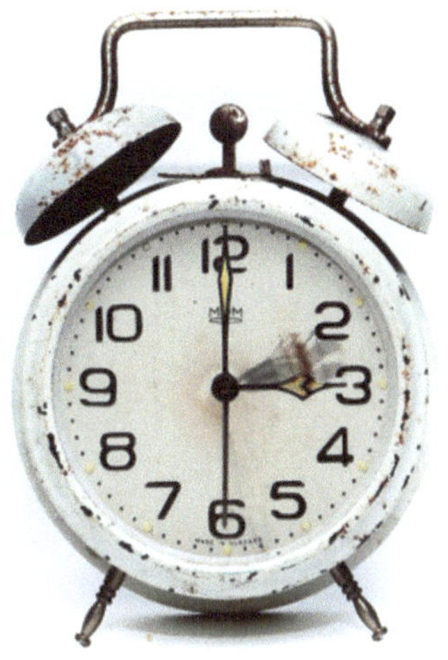

Planning your time and being conscious of the time for your activities is very vital to avoid falling into mental health issues. When you don't plan your time, you end up falling in a rush; and when you're in a rush, you end up imposing fear in your brain, thus, releasing stress hormones into your body which can affect your mental health.

Things like eating on time, drinking water on time, taking your medicine on time, sleeping on time, resting on time, and going for check-up on time are also important and not waiting when the situations become critical. Managing the time for your various activities well not only makes your engagements efficient, effective and productive, it also improves your psychological well-being.

Activity:

Get yourself a wrist watch and a planner. Set an alarm for your activities or employ someone to help you manage your time.

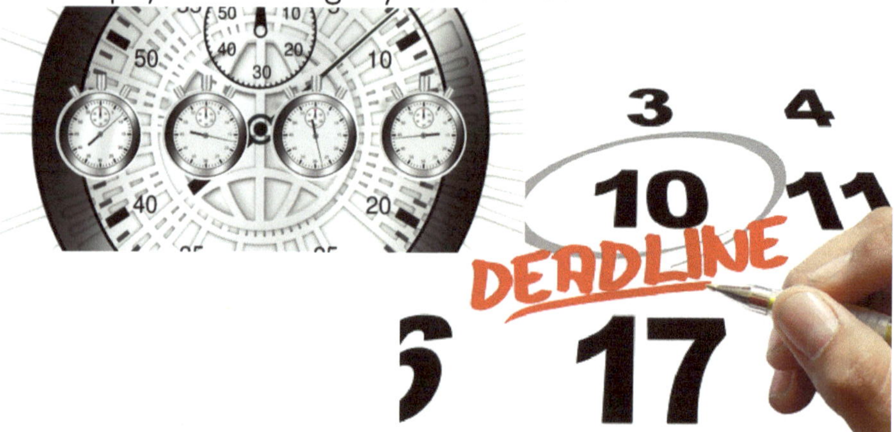

FINANCIAL MANAGEMENT

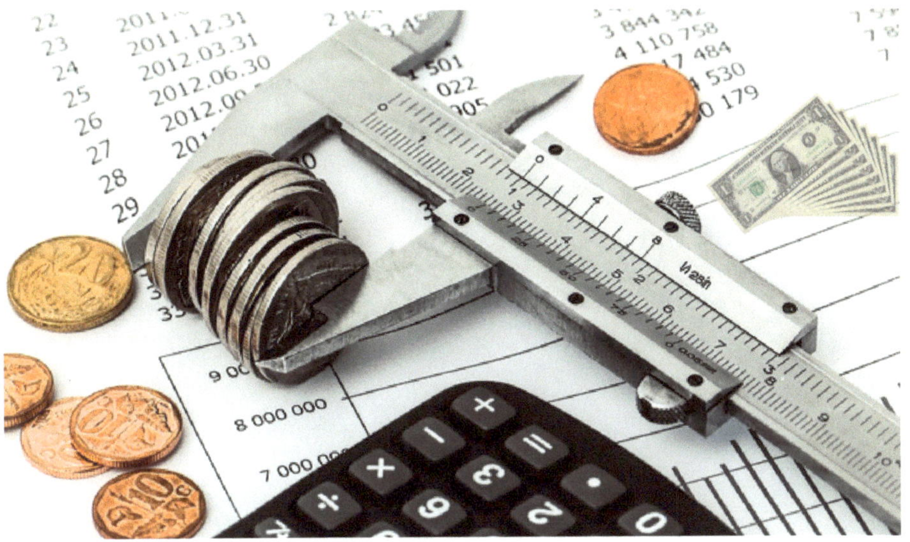

The business of money is very vital to one's psychological wellness. People think a lot about business – how to make more money, how to handle their profits, cash, credits and bonds, as well as expenses; and immediately something goes wrong their businesses, it affects them mentally, thus, leading to other negative factors.

The business of money is very vital to one's psychological wellness. People think a lot about business – how to make more money, how to handle their profits, cash, credits and bonds, as well as expenses; and immediately something goes wrong their businesses, it affects them mentally, thus, leading to other negative factors.

Activity:

Therefore, it's important to be open-minded about one's business and know that there's always profits and losses in any business. However, you need to be strategic in planning and undertaking your financial activities for more positive results.

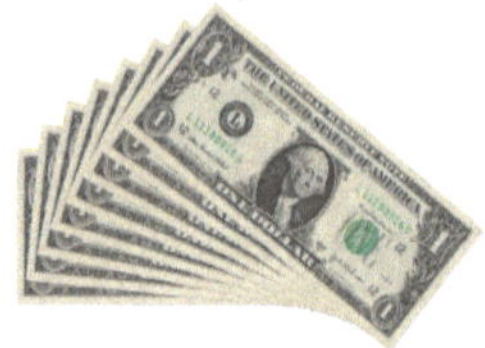
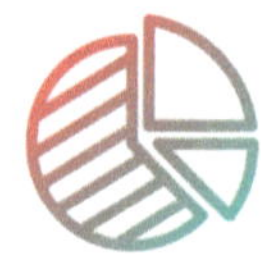
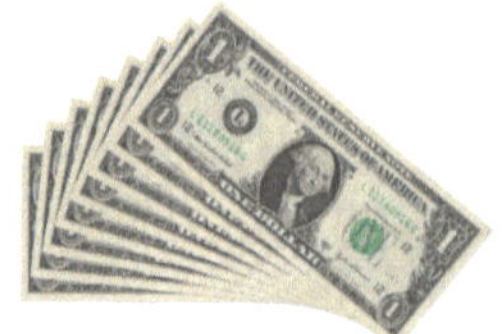

FRIENDSHIP

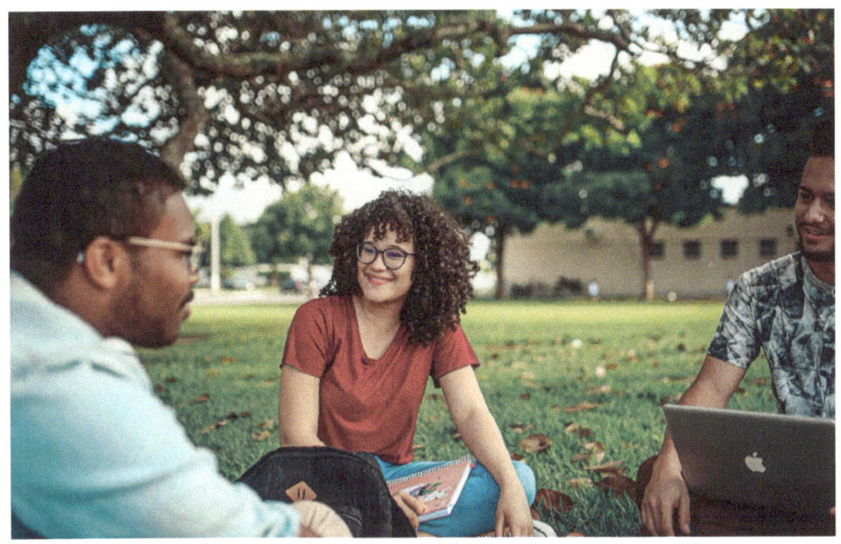

Association with like-minded people is very important to being and staying in a good mental state. Friends do provide supports which can make one to overcome or not to fall into mental health issues. However, one needs to be mindful of people one brings into his or her life; and not to be silent when one needs an advice or assistance from a friend.

Again, when you notice that your friendship with someone is becoming toxic or strangely, kindly pull off immediately for own good.

Activity:

Find people of like-minds and befriend them. Seek advice from them when necessary and know when to disconnect if the relationship starts to go south.

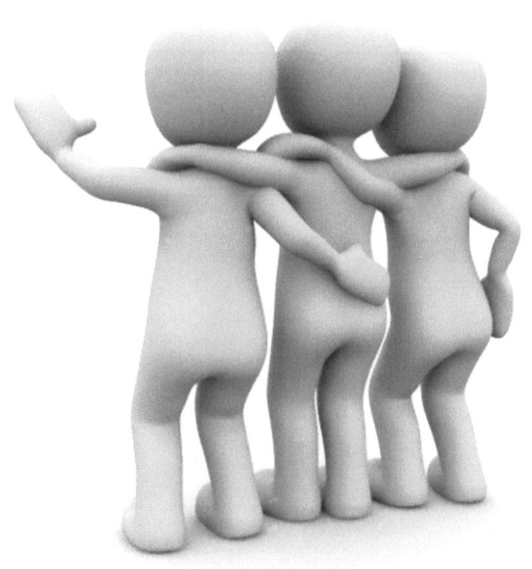

TOUR AND VACATION

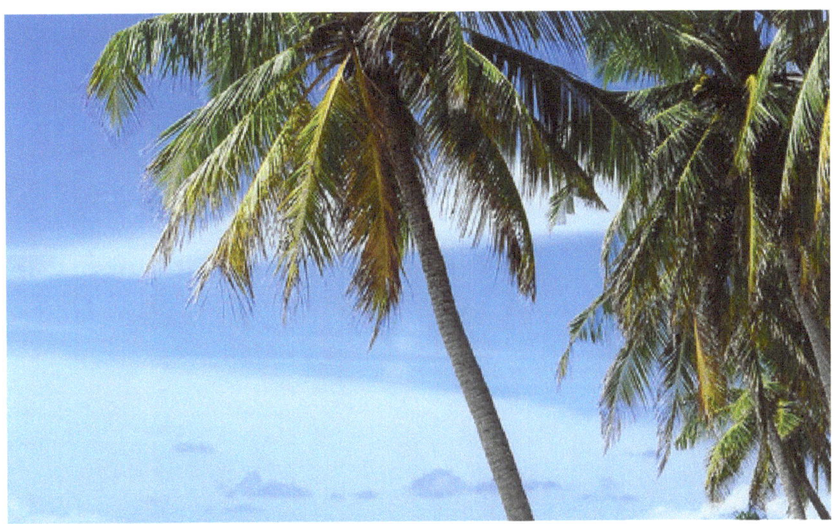

Going on vacation or a tour outside your place of abode is a good mental health strategy and adventure. People go to some of these relaxation centers like beaches, mountains, parks, zoos, museum and so on to get away from stress, negative thoughts, and improve their mental health states. They become more inspired mentally afterwards.

Activity:

Oftentimes, make a plan to tour some beautiful places and sceneries. Give it a maximum attention.

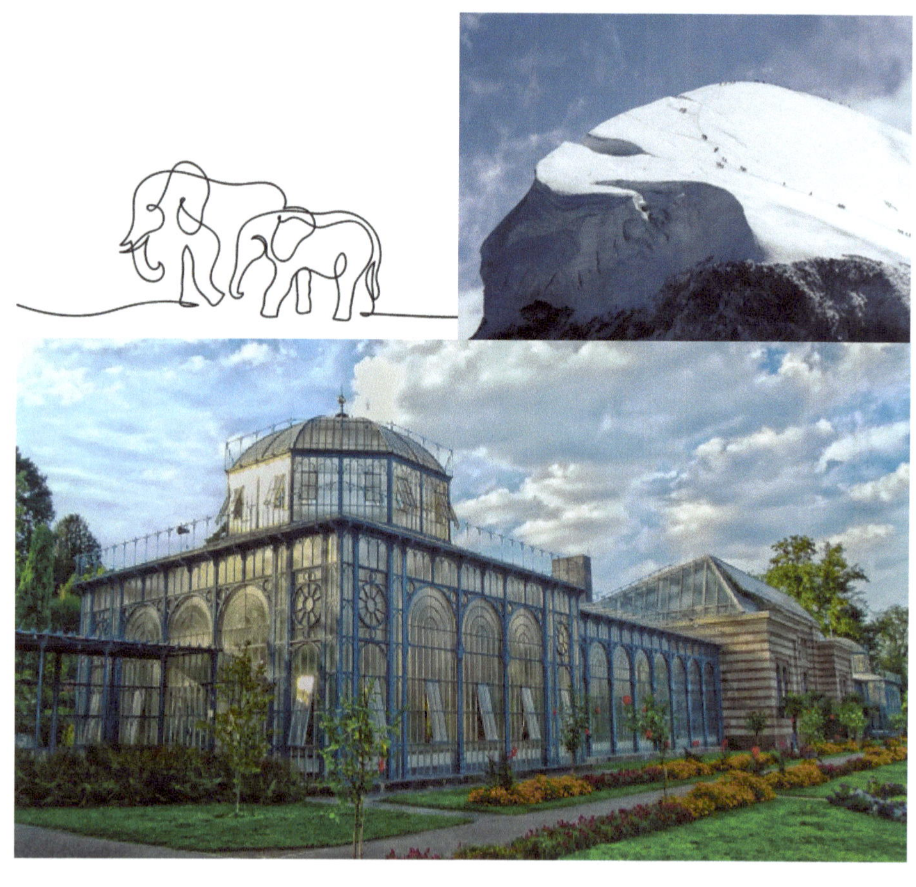

MOVIES AND TV SERIES

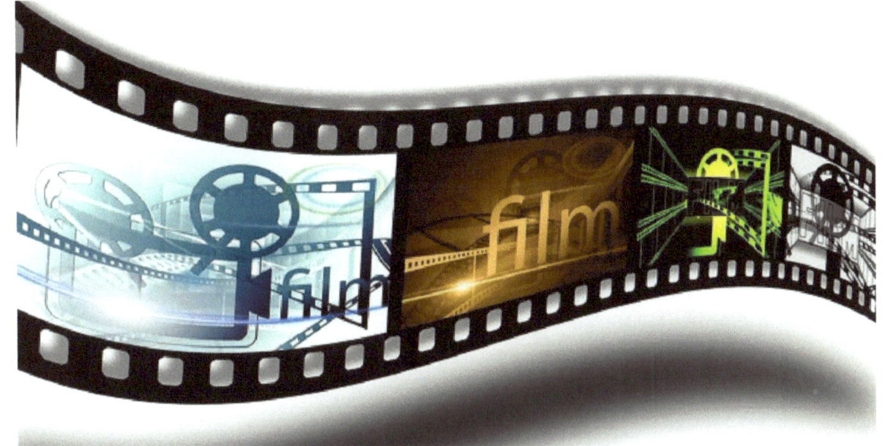

Just like music, watching movies and TV series is a great stress-relieving activity. It also drives motivation, brings good mood, relaxes the mind, in addition to educative benefits it offers. Good movies and TV series can also make one think, feel and behave better. To avoid falling into or overcome mental health issues, one needs to engage in watching movies and TV series more frequent.

Movies and TV shows can relieve your mind from bad thoughts and worries, thus, helping you overcome and not fall into mental health challenges.

Activity:

Instead of sitting down thinking about your problems - what you have and don't have, get some movies, TV series, comedic shows and watch. Go to the cinema also sometimes to see a movie or watch shows.

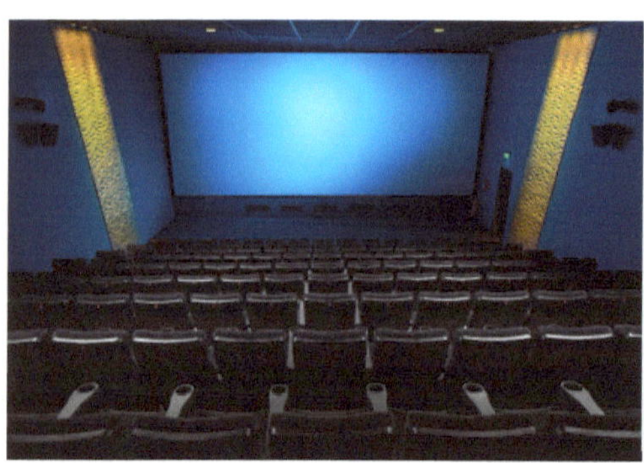
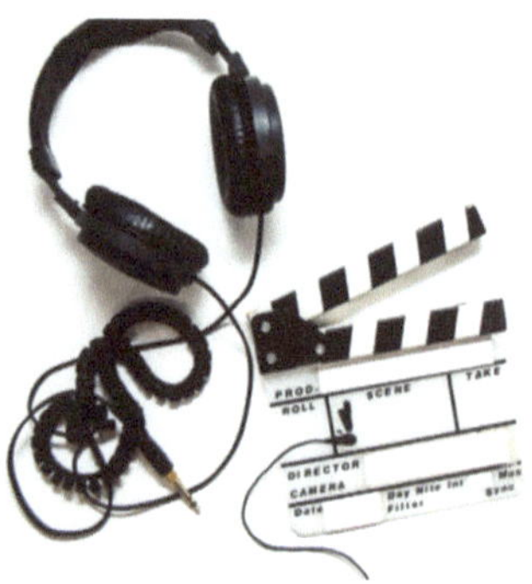

READING BOOKS AND JOURNALS

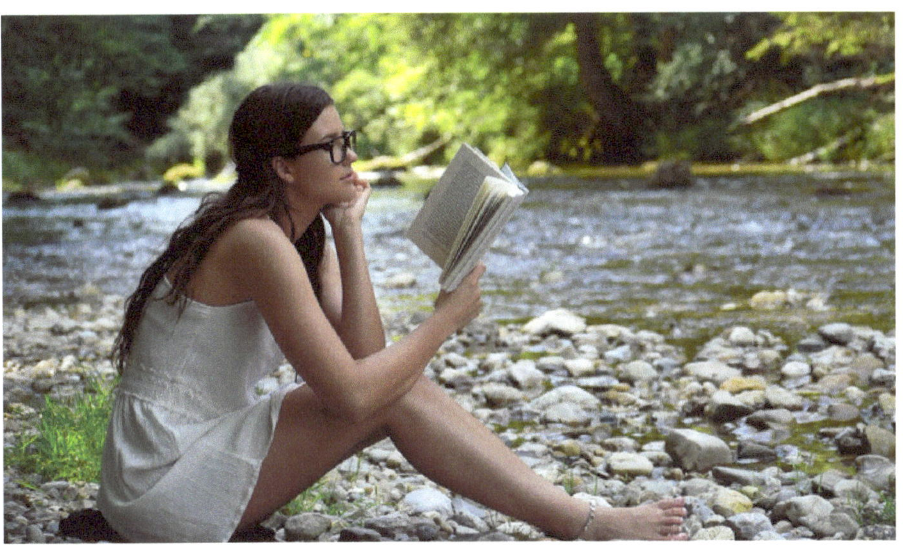

Overcoming mental health issues has something with reading good books and journals. Good books and/or journals are not only educative and life-changing, they're also therapeutic to the brain/mind. Good books like this one you're reading can make you to relax, feel motivated and help you solve your problems.

It's important you avoid bad books or journals that are demeaning or make you engage into different atrocities because they end up affecting your mental health negatively.

Activity:

From to time, get yourself good and appealing books and journals to read. Don't forget to read self-help books like this, they can change your life and improve your mental health.

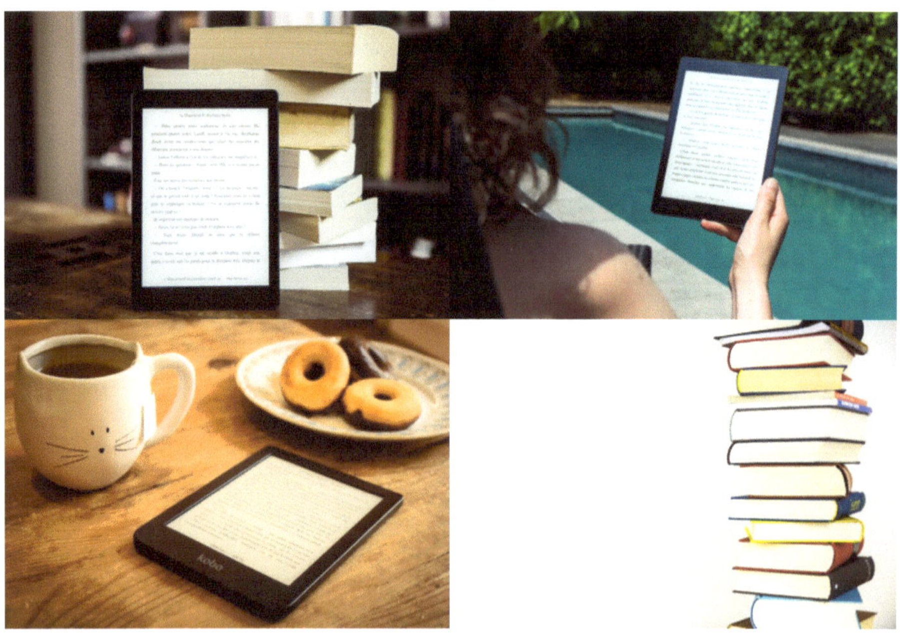

DRUG AND SUBSTANCE

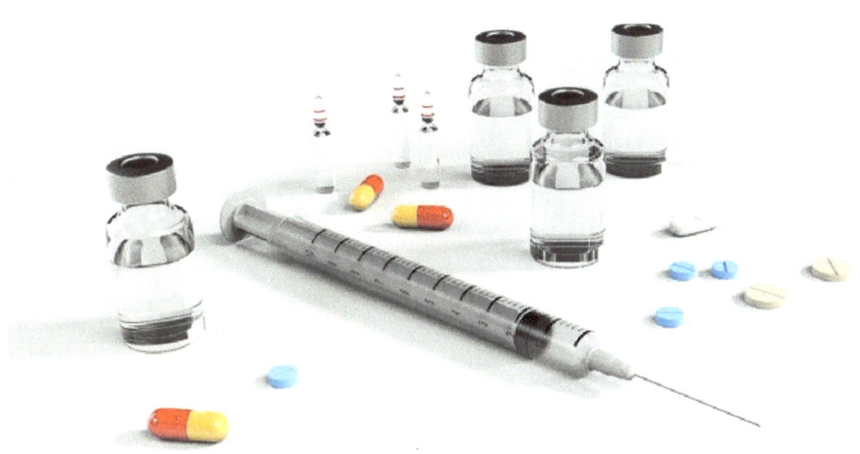

Drug and substance abuse is extremely dangerous to your overall well-being. Hard drugs like cocaine, heroine, marijuana, etc. may be used medically to perform some surgical operations, but when misused outside medical advice, then, there's a serious problem; same thing with substances like alcohols.

Despite some health importance of some of some of these drugs and substances, the abuse can lead to a lot of health problems affecting the lung, kidney, and liver diseases, also causing stroke and cancer, as well as mental health issues. When they affect one's mental health, they can cause memory loss, brain tumor, and can also push one to engage in social vices that are against the law, commit suicide or/and homicide. Therefore, taking excessive drugs and other hard substances can never be a solution to easy one's self from stress or bad feeling rather it's the road to self-destruction.

Activity:

Stop alcoholism and avoid taking or injecting yourself with hard drugs or substances. Meet a psychologist or good friends when you're feeling bad or worried.

FOOD AND DRINK

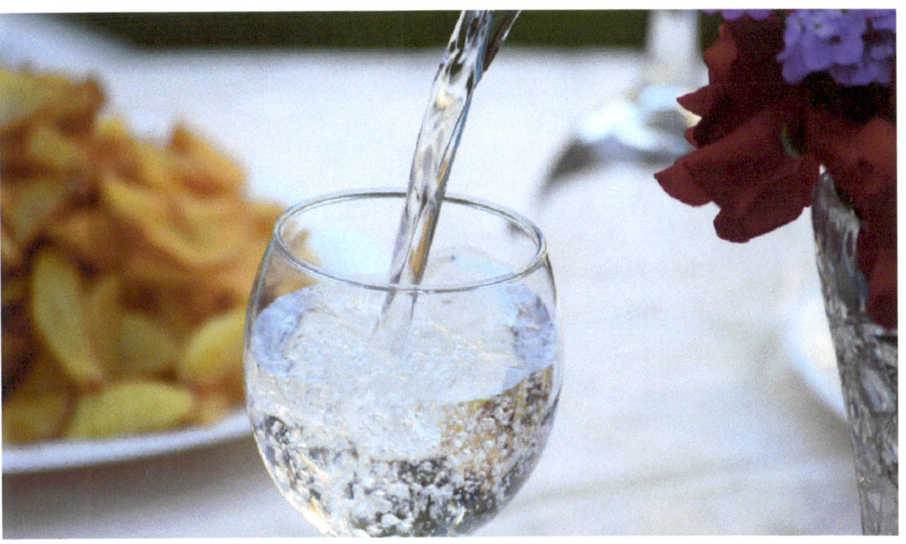

Enjoying good food and drinks can affect your mental health positively. Good food and drinks not only supply your body with the necessary supplements, vitamins and minerals needed to fight diseases and build your body energy, they also cause the production and the release of vital hormones that help in the overall psychological wellness and functionality of your brain.

The most important liquid your body needs on a regular is water, and lack of it or inadequacy of it can lead to dehydration of your system, resulting in serious mental issues. Therefore, eating good food and drinks at appropriate time can help you overcome or not fall into mental health issues.

Activity:

Eat good food and drinks, timely and always. More important, drink water and keep your body and brain hydrated. Avoid unhealthy and infested food or drinks.

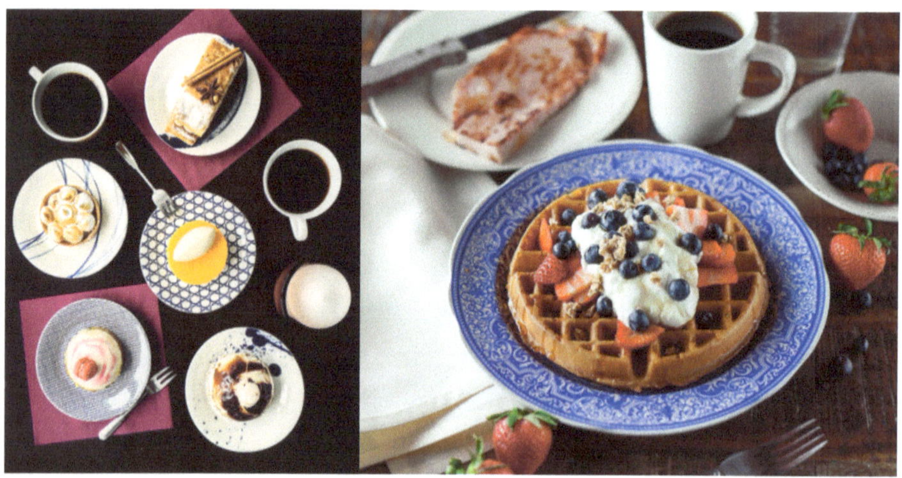

FUTURE PROSPECTS

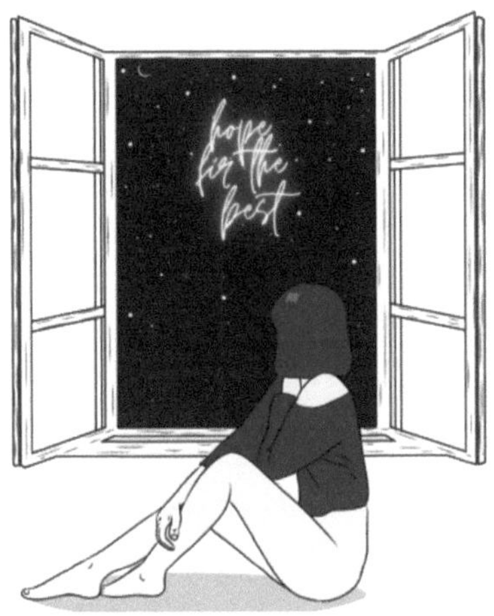

Sometimes, anxiety of what might happen in the next minute or in the future, can make one to worry and this increase one's stress, by triggering the body to generate stress-hormones, which in turn, affect one's mental health. These fears may be because of what is happening around you, what has happened to you or someone you knew in the past and bad economy; the fear of failure in marriage, in your studies and business, and the fear of not marrying, not giving birth or giving birth to a deformed baby.

The anxiety of dying untimely through disease or pandemic, dying in an accident, dying in sleep, or being killed or/and kidnapped by bad people; in addition to the fear of being attacked or raped. The prevalent ones are the fear of poverty and not achieving one's dreams in life before dying.

Activity:

Putting up proper planning, being open-minded and optimistic that you will succeed, reassuring yourself that your case will be different despite the bad happenings, and removing your mind from any negative thoughts about your future are all you need to overcome or not fall into mental health issues in this case.

YOU'RE MORE THAN A CONQUEROR

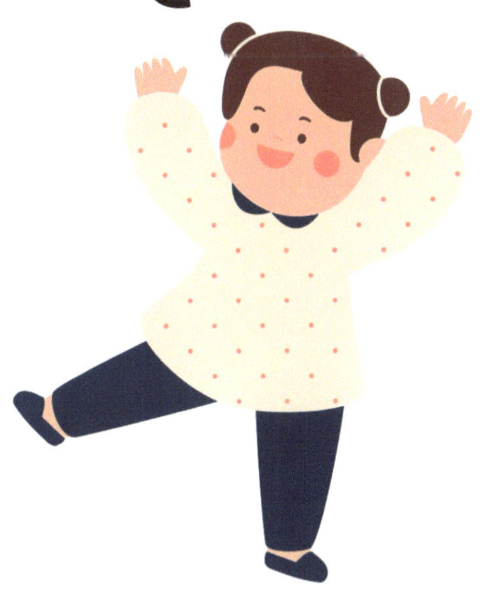

ABOUT THE AUTHOR

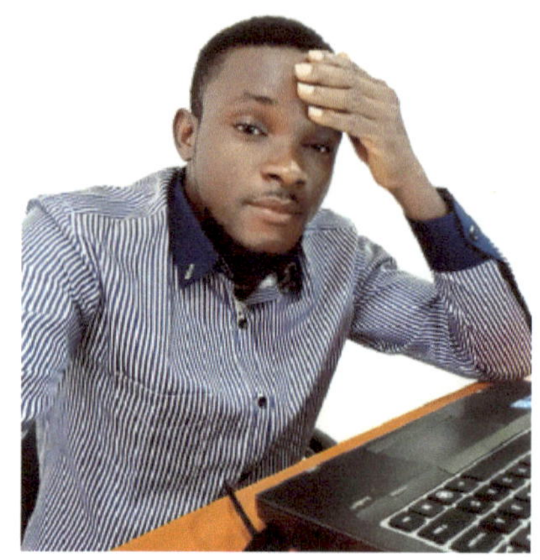

Innocent Onunkwo is an educator and a published book author from Anambra State, Nigeria. He has authored many books including A Question of Love, Taking the Boldness, The Endurance Key, Unsatisfied Lot, Profitable Inspirational Quotes for the Wise, Thoughtful Quotes that Strike the Mind, 30 Ways to Win Her Over, 30 Ways to Win Him Over, etc.

He is also a published artist (stage name: Inosky). His works are widely available. Impacting the world positively with his talents is his utmost desire.